Table of Contents

		PAGE
	INTRODUCTION	2
	PLANNING	3
	SELECTION	4
	VARIETIES	5
	PLANTING	8
	CARE	11
	PRUNING	16
	TRANSPLANTING	17
	WINTERIZING	18
	BROAD-LEAVED EVERGREENS	19
	Azaleas	19
	Holly	22
	Magnolias	23
	SHRUBS	24
	GROUNDCOVERS	29

America's / Master Gardener®

Introduction

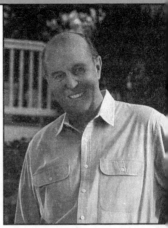

T he term "evergreen" means what it says - the plant will keep its foliage year-round, and in most cases, the foliage is green. There are, however, many evergreens that have 2 faces — a summer face and a winter one. These plants are green in summer but turn a beautiful burgundy color in winter. So when selecting plants for your landscape, buy ones that are as attractive in winter as they are in summer.

Contrary to popular belief, not all evergreens have needles. Many have leaves like any flowering shrub, and they are called broad-leaved evergreens. Many in this group, like rhododendrons and azaleas, also have 2 faces, the difference being that they produce foliage in winter and flowers in spring. With a little bit of planning and a lot of imagination, you can make quite a masterpiece out of your yarden.

This booklet is your first step towards creating that masterpiece. I'll tell you how to select, plant and care for your evergreens using common sense and common household items.

If you have an evergreen, shrub, or groundcover question, why don't you call me **"On the Garden Line"** Saturday mornings from 8:00 a.m. - 10:00 a.m. EST, on your local Mutual Broadcasting Station. The toll-free number is **1-800-634-3881**.

Also, for more comprehensive information, please refer to one of my other full-size books:

**Plants Are Still Like People
Jerry Baker's Flowering Garden
The Impatient Gardener**

or pick up a copy of **America's Gardening Newsletter, "On The Garden Line®,"** which is also jam-packed with timely tips, tricks and tonics on lawn, garden and house plant care.

PLANNING

A good, workable plan doesn't have to be a complicated work of art by a landscape architect. A piece of scratch paper or a grocery bag cut open will do nicely.

First, survey your property. Pace off the length and width if you do not already know them. Next, pace off the distance from your property lines to your house, and other building locations. Then continue by adding the walkways, driveway, fences and existing flower beds or other gardens. On your plan, you must indicate where the downspouts are, any low spots that can or do hold water, and existing shade trees. Also, show the size of the shadow they cast and for what period of time each day.

I have found that using colors makes identification much easier. I use green for trees, gray for walk and driveways, black for buildings, brown for gardens and beds, chartreuse for wet spots, and blue for water, ponds or streams. Be sure to code the colors in the margins for quick and easy identification.

Also indicate all doors and windows. The last thing to do is to indicate which direction is north on the plan with a small red "N" and an arrow pointing north. The end? Not by a long shot! What's next? Selection.

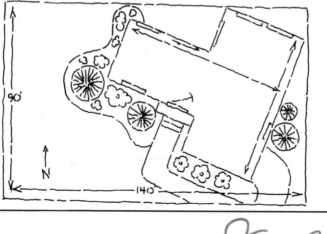

SELECTION

There are many things that you should remember when you're selecting evergreens, shrubs, and groundcovers. First and foremost, pick plants that will complement your home, not hide it.

Choose colors that will not clash with the brick or siding. Pick shapes that will not make your house look taller or shorter, wider or narrower. Choose plants that grow low in front of low windows, so they don't shut out the view. Choose taller plants for corners, to break the sharp edges.

But where can you find all of this information? **Your mailbox!** That's right, if you will just send away for several of the mail order nursery catalogues that are offered in any of the national magazines, soon the Mail Order Nurseryman's Association will be beating a path to your door! Most catalogues are free; some have a nominal charge, but they are worth the money. These catalogues are an encyclopedia of garden information and background on the guests (evergreens, that is) that you are going to invite to share your little corner of the world. Most include lots and lots of pictures that make your decisions easier.

When the catalogues arrive, look them over and decide what you want where. Then pencil them in on your plans (don't use pen or crayon for this because plans are always subject to change).

Your next step should be to visit your local nursery or garden center that specializes in these materials. Chose a reputable retailer, one that guarantees his nursery stock. The nurseryman will gladly go over your plan, point out a change or two, offer suggestions and help you figure out costs.

You may have had a hard time deciding which members of the large evergreen family you want to bring home with you. In the next section, I discuss some of the more common members of both branches of the family — the broad-leaved and the coniferous evergreens — to help you decide.

VARIETIES

CONIFERS or narrow-leaved evergreens come in all shapes and sizes, just like the members of any other large family. Some are tall and slender, others are tall and pyramid-shaped, while still others are very short and squat. Be sure you know what shape a young evergreen will grow into before you plant it.

ARBORVITAE have been popular in America for a long time. They root easily, grow quickly, and are available in several sizes and shapes. There are two types of Arborvitae — the native White-cedar or American Arborvitae, and Oriental Arborvitae. Both have flat, scale-like leaves that look very much like the fonds of certain ferns, and small, dried capsules as fruit.

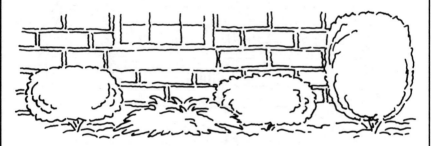

THE DOUGLAS FIRS are very handsome members of the ever-green family who are too often neglected. Nursery plants often look unimpressive, but as the trees get older, they develop a symmetrical pyramidal shape and bear their branches well down to the ground when grown in the open.

JUNIPERS form one of the largest branches on the evergreen family tree. There are more than 170 different species and varieties, so your choice is limited only by your needs. Junipers range in size from creeping groundcovers to full-sized trees. They'll do well in hot, dry, sunny locations and in urban areas; locations some of their more temperamental relatives wouldn't tolerate. Most can be pruned easily and some can be trimmed into hedge form. They all prefer soil that is not too acidic.

🌲 VARIETIES

HEMLOCKS have small, soft needles, pendulous branches and tiny intricate cones that are no more than 2" long. Trees are tall, dark green and pyramidal.

There are 6 main species of hemlocks used for landscaping. All are shallow rooted, which makes them easy to transplant. All can be trimmed into excellent hedges, and all grow well in shade, unlike many of their sun-loving relatives.

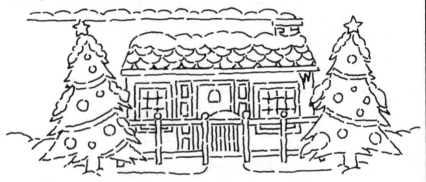

PINES make up a large and impressive group in the evergreen family, and they are the most popular ornamental evergreen.

Most pines grow in tree form, but there are a few shrubs among them. Pine needles are long and grow in clusters of 2, 3 or 5 bound together by a membranous sheath. Cones vary in size and shape from species to species.

Pines are wonderful problem solvers. You can find varieties that will be perfectly happy in poor or sandy soil.

SPRUCES are not among my favorite evergreens. Few of them grow up into worthwhile adults - most lose their lower branches or become ragged and uneven. Because they take up a lot of room, they can only be used as prominent specimen plants.

All spruces except the dwarf varieties grow into rigid, pyramidal trees with single trunks. Needles are sharp and pointed.

YEWS are unique among the narrow-leaved evergreens. They make excellent landscaping plants since they grow well in most soils, and can adapt themselves to either sun or shade. They don't even seem to mind pruning, so they can be trimmed into beautiful hedge and topiary designs, or confined to a small growing space for a long time. The hybrid varieties come in many different sizes and shapes, ranging from a dwarf, almost prostrate form, to narrowly columnar shapes.

CEDARS have small clustered needles and large erect cones. All grow into very large trees. They are not hardy where winters are severe. The only true cedars are the Deodar Cedar, the Atlas Cedar, and the Cedar of Lebanon.

FALSE CYPRESS are trees and shrubs with flat, spray-like foliage and very small cones. All members of the Cypress clan are very tender and delicate. They thrive only in very temperate climates. The most common varieties are:

Lawson False Cypress - to 120'. Grows best in mild climates with lots of moisture. Limited to use on the West Coast. Shrub, dwarf and yellow varieties are available.

Hinoki False Cypress - to 120'. Hardier than Lawson False Cypress. Slow-growing, pyramidal tree with glossy, scale-like green leaves. Dwarf, shrubby and yellow varieties are available.

Sawara False Cypress - to 150'. Hardier than Lawson False Cypress. Narrow, pyramidal tree with loose, open growth pattern. Tends to lose lower branches. Varieties with feathery silvery foliage, yellow foliage, and dwarf and compact growth habits, are available.

Italian Cypress - tall, spire-like trees that can be grown in California and in many of the southern states.

Arizona Cypress - narrow, pyramidal tree with green or bluish-gray foliage. Does well in southern states. Tolerates cold better than other cypress.

PLANTING

Most folks think that all there is to planting an evergreen is to dig a hole, drop in a bush, refill the hole with soil and watch the bush grow. When planting any living plant, you must handle the plant as delicately as possible. The precise location, as well as the permanent angle, should be well thought out.

The planting procedure actually begins before you ever bring the evergreen home. By this I mean that you must first investigate the soil conditions where you are going to ask these plants to grow. Most evergreens are grown in light, loose soil, or growing mixes with good drainage. Therefore, I suggest that when you are preparing your evergreen beds, you add liberal quantities of 60-40 gravel to the existing soil if it is heavy. Sandy soil needs no preparation.

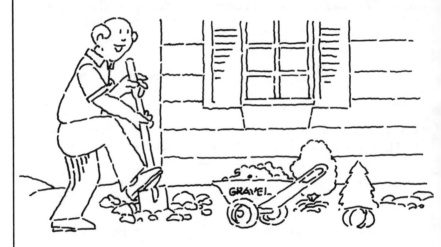

In heavy clay soil, it is important that you determine your water table and the direction of the water's surface flow. Many an unsuspecting gardener has placed a plant in a spot that displayed it at its best, only to find that when it rained, the water from the downspout or the surface water from the grade flowed right over the top of the evergreen, the hole filled up with water and the plant died.

Evergreens come in three basic containers: **balled-in-burlap, metal containers,** and **plantable paper-pulp pots.** The container doesn't make much difference. The plantable container, however, is fast becoming the most popular because the average home gardener can plant it with the least amount of fuss and plant shock. The metal container is rather cumbersome, and the plant must be removed from the container, which means cutting the sides of the can which can result in a few minor cuts and scratches. Soil is often shaken loose from the roots in the process, exposing them to the air, which can cause damage to the plant.

The balled-in-burlap is an excellent container, but it is fast becoming a thing of the past thanks to automation, increased production, and a lack of ballers. A good baller has the skill and speed of any good journeyman. How he handles the plant when it is dug determines whether or not it lives in your yard.

THE RIDE HOME

You have just selected and paid for your plants. Next comes the ride home. This may just be a one-way ride if it is not done properly.

Whenever it can be avoided, plants that are in containers should not be laid down on their sides in a trunk or on a back seat. This tends to crush the sides, loosen the soil and expose the roots. Balled-in-burlap plants should not be allowed to roll around and bang the sides for the same reasons. Set the plant containers upright and brace them. Block balled plants to keep them from rolling.

More evergreens lose their lives on driveways or in garages than any other place. Once you have made the plan, selected the plants, and purchased the materials, take your time! But make sure you plant your evergreens the day you bring them home!

JUST DIG A HOLE

No one likes to live in cramped quarters, and this is especially true of evergreens. If the planting hole is too small and cramped, the new visitor will be uncomfortable, its growth will be stunted, and it will soon become ill. I was always taught to dig a hole half as wide as the width of the container. This is referred to as digging a $10.00 hole for a $5.00 plant.

Your evergreens should be planted only 1" to 1-1/2" deeper than they were in the nursery. If you plant them too deep, you might smother the roots.

FILL IT UP FILTERED

Almost without exception, all evergreens love loose, well-drained soil. If your evergreens do not have first-class living conditions, soon they will not be living. It's as simple as that.

What can you do? First, you should determine if you have good drainage. The hole is now dug and you are reasonably certain that the plant will sit straight and level. Get out the garden hose and fill the hole with water (but don't wash away the sides or alter the base). Watch closely. If the water has not subsided in a few minutes, you have a drainage problem. To correct this, dig a narrow trench, the depth of the hole, on an angle parallel with the downward grade of the property and fill it with gravel. If, on the other hand, the water runs through the hole like a sieve, you can line the hole with clay loam to hold some moisture.

In the case of the balled-in-burlap plant, after you have half filled the hole, it will be necessary to cut the twine at the top of the ball and where it is bound around the trunk.

Do not, I repeat, **do not feed** newly planted shrubs right away. Let them get used to the soil and their new neighbors for a couple of weeks, and then give them a light snack of any one of the fish emulsion fertilizers. Then feed them again at the end of the month with a low-nitrogen, dry garden food, like 4-12-4 or 5-10-5, to stimulate root growth. In the meantime, cover up the roots with a 2" deep mulch of wood chips that extends all the way out to the ends of the bottom branches.

CARE

ost folks who plant evergreens take them for granted. If you want to get along with your evergreens, you've got to feed them. They need food, and they aren't capable of foraging for themselves like their ancestors who grew free in the woods in a thick, rich layer of natural organic mulch that fed them continuously.

FEEDING

Write this on your garden calendar: feed your evergreens in February, April, and June. Never, ever feed them after August 15 if you live in snow country. If you live in the warmer areas, feed them in August and October, too.

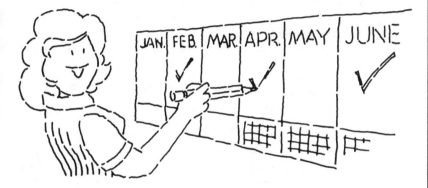

You should feed all of your evergreens with the same dry fertilizer you use on your lawn, except for "Weed & Feed". Feed at the rate of one-half pound per foot of height. Sprinkle the food over the top of the wood chip mulch underneath your evergreens, then watch the difference. The plants will be singing the number 1 song on the Tree Top Parade: "What a Difference a Meal Makes."

You can also feed using any of the liquid fish emulsions. Why not use dry one time and liquid the next? The cartridge feeders also do a nice job.

America's / Master Gardener®

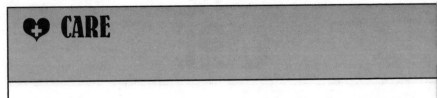

If some of your evergreens are in out-of-the-way places, you can use well-rotted manure as both mulch and fertilizer. Spread a layer 2" to 3" deep over the area beneath the spread of the branches.

Trees use commercial fertilizer best when it is spread in a 2' to 3' wide circular band below the outer tips of the branches. Water the fertilizer in.

When large trees begin to look undernourished, make a ring of holes beneath the outer tips of the branches with a tree auger or crowbar. The holes should be 6" to 8" deep and 2' apart. Place a handful of fertilizer in each hole and add water to dissolve it. You don't need to plug the holes - they'll let air and water to the roots.

WATERING

Your evergreens need an occasional drink. It's true that evergreens growing in a forest need only rainfall, but forest soil is always covered with a deep, moisture-holding mulch of leaves and leaf mold.

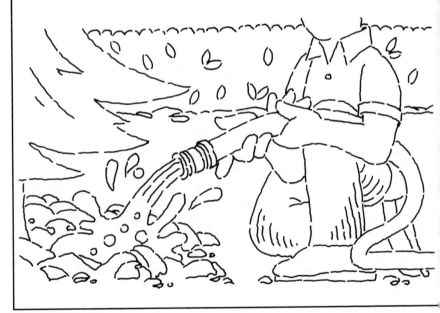

Mulching your evergreens will help, but they still have to compete with the lawn and other plants for moisture. Also, the roots of young plants don't go beyond the root ball for several years after planting, so their feeding area is limited. Water all young evergreens regularly, at least until they become well established. Mother Nature should be able to handle things on her own from then on.

When watering, remove the nozzle from the hose and let the water soak into the soil until no more can be absorbed. Don't be satisfied with a light sprinkling — shallow watering encourages the development of surface roots at the expense of main roots. Even in dry weather, 1 thorough watering every 10 to 14 days should be sufficient.

It's also a good idea to give your evergreens a shower every now and then, especially during dry, dusty weather. This shower will wash off dust, drown certain insects and give your evergreens a brighter complexion. Remember, a clean face is a happy face!

DISEASES

In early spring (or late winter in the west and south), begin your evergreen health-care program. Bathe them with this tonic in your 20 gal. hose-end sprayer.

1 cup liquid dish soap

1 cup chewing tobacco juice*

1 cup antiseptic mouthwash

fill the balance of the sprayer jar with warm water

Wash inside and out, over and under; don't miss any spots! Viruses and fungus diseases are the result of poor hygiene, airborne silt, dust and various pollutants that settle on the foliage and needles. These frequent showers keep the pores and cells open, and allow photosynthesis to take place in a normal manner. It is absolutely imperative that you bathe your evergreens at least once a month, and more often in heavy smog or industrial areas.

*To make chewing tobacco juice, place 3 fingers of chewing tobacco in an old nylon stocking and soak it in a gallon of hot water until the mixture is dark brown.

America's / Master Gardener®

Fungicides are the chemicals used to control and cure the diseases that attack your evergreens. Every manufacturer of lawn and garden products has at least one broad spectrum fungicide that will solve most problems. These chemicals will not restore the appearance of your evergreens after an injury caused by a virus; they only prevent the spread of the disease. So once the damage is done, don't expect miracles from the fungicides.

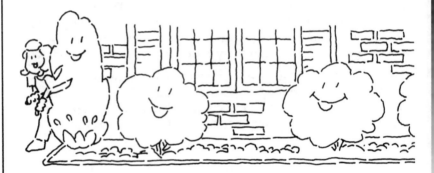

MULCHING

A good layer of mulch will hold down weeds, act as a source of food, and contain moisture. A good-looking mulch enhances the appearance of the plant itself and lets it show off. There are many to choose from; some are better than others because they do not attract rodents. I like hardwood chips, and redwood and pine bark. I do not particularly like cocoa bean shells, buckwheat hulls and straw because they attract insects and mice.

Stone chips are also an attractive mulch that holds down weeds and contains moisture. The assortment of stone materials is limitless, from hard coal chips to pea gravel. Many garden centers now offer a type of coated stone of bright colors that is extremely attractive. With some imagination, you can use these stones to create many unusual and eye-catching effects. A clean, neat well-trimmed and mulched garden will display healthy evergreens at their best.

INSECT CONTROL

We are right back to the bath routine. Bugs have eyes, mouths, noses and very delicate stomachs. When you bathe your yarden, the bugs that are around get the soap-tobacco juice-mouthwash mixture in their eyes, up their noses and in their mouths. If they're still alive, they'll soon move on. New bugs stopping by for a snack or to set up housekeeping soon discover the food in "dis here plaz" is not very tasty, and their stomachs are constantly upset. So they too move on.

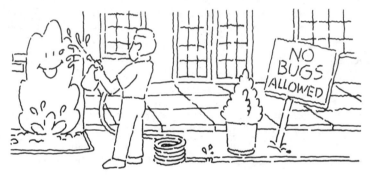

Insects have a great communication network, and they will soon pass the word along about your place. Not all bugs fly, as you know, nor do they all like the taste of foliage. Some prefer the tender young roots. To discourage these underground visitors, poke a series of hole into the soil beneath the branches and hose down this area with the same solution. Not all of the bugs will give up quite this easily, and it may be necessary to turn to the chemical controls. When this becomes necessary, use only the manufacturer's recommended chemical strength to do the job. I have found that Malathion will pretty much take care of the chewing and sucking insects, and Dursban ends the underground problems.

I will make a brief comment about combining 2 or more chemicals for a stronger wallop. Watch out, you're playing with fire. Always follow the manufacturer's recommendations!

Jerry Baker

America's / Master Gardener®

PRUNING

Trimming can begin in the warmer areas in March, and as soon as the snow disappears in the rest of the country. As new growth appears, continue trimming to keep your evergreens looking neat and natural. Electric hedge trimmers work fine and save a lot of work. If you properly plant, feed, mulch and care for your evergreens, they will grow tall, wide, and full.

When pruning any plant, your tools must be sharp. You can trim evergreens as often as you like, and you should do so periodically to contain them so they don't grow over the sidewalk or cover the windows. When trimming yews and junipers, you cannot "invert your trim." I mean that your design can be perpendicular or flared, but cannot be cut inward because when you do this, the upper branches cast a shadow and shut out the sun. When this occurs, the needles will begin to drop.

NEEDLE DROP

Needle drop seems to upset many a home gardener when he is not aware of what's happening. Most evergreens naturally shed their older, central needles in fall, and this is no cause for alarm. It is when the outside needles begin to drop that you should worry.

Every so often, you should shake your evergreens. Go ahead, give them a good slap on the back! This is like scratching your dog's stomach, and will help shake out some of the natural needle drop that occurs in most evergreens.

When evergreens begin to look thin-haired, it is usually because of 1 of 2 things: insects or poor trimming. First, check for insects. If you can't see them, get a sheet of white paper, place it under several different branches, and shake them. Then look closely at the paper. If bugs are the problem, you will see them scoot around the paper. If there is no sign of insects, look over your shrub carefully and ask these questions: Are all of the sides getting full sun? Did I use dull shears and injure the foliage? Did I cut too far back and expose coarse inner branches? If any of your answers are "yes", then shame on you!

TRANSPLANTING

In most areas, August is generally an excellent month to move evergreens. Most evergreens have finished their growth for the current year and have set their buds for the next. From then on, most of the plants' efforts are concentrated on root growth.

Of course, you can't just dig them up willy-nilly. You must dig them with a good root ball and transplant them correctly. Since the soil may be dry, it is a good idea to soak the soil around the plants a day or 2 in advance. This keeps the soil from falling off of the roots in all but the sandiest of locations.

Dig your new hole one-half wider than the root ball you intend to dig and as much or deeper. In the bottom, make sure that there is not less than a foot of good soil to which you have added a half-and-half mixture of dried cow manure and moistened peat moss.

Now you are ready to dig up the evergreen. Cut down around it as deeply as you can, undercutting as you go until you have completely severed the ball from the earth. Next, lift the tree out, not by the trunk but by prying and lifting with your shovel.

If your plant is relatively small, you can slide it to its new home on the shovel. If not, try sliding it on a piece of cardboard, canvas or burlap bag. This is much easier than carrying it and it protects the ball from breaking.

When you get it into the hole, fill one-half with an improved soil as above, tamp and flood with water. When this has drained away, complete the filling but do not tamp, leaving a basin around the plant to hold water.

Next, cover the soil around the plant and a foot or 2 beyond with an inch or 2 of any good mulch like shredded bark to retain moisture. Finally, spray the foliage thoroughly with CloudCover® to prevent wilting and drying out before the roots get established.

America's / Master Gardener®

❄ WINTERIZING

To get ready for winter, first spray all of your evergreens with CloudCover® in late fall to prevent unnecessary water loss and winter kill. This will save you time, money and aggravation next spring.

Evaporation through the foliage occurs in winter as well as in summer. If the roots dry out, there will be little moisture in the plants and foliage burning may occur during periods of bright sunshine. Therefore, give your evergreens a thorough watering in late fall just before the ground freezes.

Spread extra mulch around your evergreens. For a winter mulch, it's best to use materials which don't pack down tightly, such as straw, ground cornstalks, or buckwheat hulls. If the plants are exposed to the wind, place slats or boards on the mulch to hold it in place.

Try to keep snow from piling up on small or shrubby evergreens, since branches and twigs can break under the weight of a heavy snow. Some evergreens, such as arborvitae and junipers, often have multiple stems. To prevent snow from bending these down and breaking them apart, tie the tops together with strips of cloth or nylon stockings.

The heavy branches of mature trees sometime break under the weight of ice or snow. If possible, shake off the ice or snow or prop up the branch with a sturdy board. And do not throw snow or ice that has salt mixed in with it on or under your evergreens!

If some of your evergreens are tender or not well adapted to your area, it's a good idea to erect a shade to protect them from wind and bright sun, both of which cause burning. To make a shade, drive wooden stakes into the ground and staple a piece of burlap between them. If wind is the main threat, place the screen between the plant and the direction of the prevailing wind. If the plant is growing in full sun, erect screens on the south and west sides to protect against the hot afternoon sun.

BROAD-LEAVED
Evergreens

Broad-leaved evergreens bear little resemblance to their narrow-leaved distant cousins. There's not much family resemblance within the broad-leaved clan either, and most of the plants that are "evergreen" in the South and in mild areas along the West Coast are not evergreen in the rest of the country.

Since broad-leaved evergreens make up such a large, loose-knit family, I'm not going to try to introduce you to all the members. I'll stick to a few of the more common, generally hardy types, and leave it up to you to make friends with the rest.

AZALEAS

Azaleas and rhododendrons are very close relatives and therefore, they should be treated equally. I'm going to talk about azaleas, but everything I tell you can be applied to rhododendrons as well.

Azaleas vary in their ability to withstand heat and cold. Ask your local nurseryman which varieties adapt to your area best.

Buy sturdy, well-branched plants that are about 16" tall. Smaller plants are more likely to be injured in winter. Plants shorter than 8" should be grown in a coldframe for a year or 2 before setting outdoors.

It's best to plant azaleas when they're dormant—in early spring before new leaves start to grow in the North and from fall to early spring in the South.

Azaleas are too fond of showing off to do well in heavy shade. You can grow them in full sun or moderate shade, but they'll do best in alternating sun and shade. One of the best places to plant azaleas is under a tall, deep-rooted tree, like an oak or pine, where they'll get a nice mixture of sun and shade. Don't plant azaleas under shallow-rooted trees that will steal moisture and nutrients from the soil. If you want to plant azaleas around a building, put them on the north or east side where they'll be protected from the hot afternoon sun.

Mature rhododendrons spread to about 8' in diameter; mature azaleas spread 4' to 6'. Space them so they won't be crowded. For a mass of blooms, set young plants close together and transplant alternate ones to other locations as they become crowded.

Prepare the planting site several weeks before planting. Dig individual holes at least 18" wide and 12" deep. For bed planting, prepare the soil to a depth of about 1'.

Azaleas like acidic soil that holds moisture but is well drained. Adding peat moss, 1- to 2-year-old oak leaves, or forest leafmold increases soil acidity, and improves the water-holding capacity of sandy soils and the drainage of clay soils. Spread a 5" layer of organic matter over the beds and work in to a depth of 6". For individual holes, mix the soil removed with an equal amount of organic matter. Level the soil unless it is heavy, or unless your have frequent hard rains in your area. In either case, leave the soil mounded to improve surface drainage.

Carefully remove the plants from non-plantable containers and set them in the holes. Don't remove the burlap from balled plants—just cut the twine after you set it in the hole.

Before filling up the hole, make sure the plant is set no deeper than it was at the nursery. If it is, pack soil under it. If the roots are buried too deeply, they won't be able to breathe properly.

Press the soil around the rootball. After the hole is full, soak the soil thoroughly so it will settle in around the roots.

As soon as the plants are set, spread a 2" to 5" mulch of oak leaves, peat moss, pine needles or leaf mold on the soil around them. Add new mulching material every spring.

Azaleas usually don't need much pruning, but if you want to shape them or reduce their size, you can do so with a clear conscience. Azaleas will tolerate severe pruning. Pruned plants won't have as many blooms the next season, but after that, they'll bloom more profusely than ever.

Be sure to give your azaleas plenty of water during their first 2 years in their new home. Give each plant about 2 gallons of water every 10 days from spring to late fall. Wait 10 days after a heavy rain before resuming your watering program. After this, rainfall is usually adequate (except during prolonged dry periods), unless azaleas are planted under eaves.

For fertilizer to be effective, it should be in liquid form and should reach the feeding roots which are located under and beyond the outside branches.

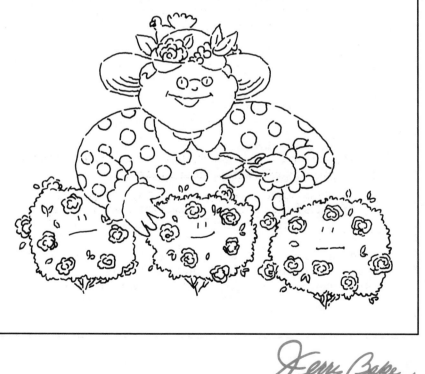

HOLLY

Many different types of holly are available, including both shrub and tree forms. Some are not evergreen in all parts of the country, and some will not grow well in certain areas. If you live in the Southwest, the Rocky Mountains or the Plains States, you shouldn't invite hollies to your home—they will be very short-lived guests. Elsewhere, ask your nurseryman which hollies are best suited for your area.

Hollies are happiest in neutral to slightly acidic, well-drained loam, but can be grown in other types of soil as well. Plant, mulch, and water hollies the same as magnolias.

The best time to **fertilize** hollies is in mid-March or late fall. Use a fertilizer specially prepared for acid-loving, broad-leaved evergreens. For trees with a trunk 1/2" or less, use 1/2 pound of fertilizer; for larger trees, use 1 to 2 pounds per inch of trunk diameter.

You may not need to **prune** your holly at all, but if you want to remove dead or damaged branches, do so during the dormant season. I like to prune hollies at Christmas so I can use the branches for decoration.

But don't overprune! If a branch is cut back to the trunk or if a twig is cut back to the branch, new growth may not appear. Coat all wounds over 1/2" in diameter with a tree dressing.

Only female hollies produce berries—and then only if they have been pollinated. If you have a holly that refuses to produce berries, then you have one of the following problems:
- The plant is male.
- The plant is female, but has no male nearby to pollinate its flowers, or no nearby male flowers at the same time as the female.
- The plant is too young to flower.
- Late frosts or cold weather injured the flowers.
- Cold, rainy weather prevented insects from spreading pollen.

MAGNOLIAS

MAGNOLIAS

Two kinds of magnolias are grown in this country—native and Asian. Only one of the native magnolias—the Southern magnolia—is evergreen in areas outside the South. All Asian magnolias are deciduous. You may want to try some of the non-evergreen magnolias, especially some of the Asians with pink, red or purple blooms.

The Southern magnolia grows 30' to 50' tall. You've certainly seen its blossoms—if not in person, in movies about the Old South. They are white, very large—6" to 10" across—and have a strong, sweet fragrance. The leaves are dark green and shiny.

Early spring is the **best time to plant** magnolias. Buy 2-year-old plants, either in containers or balled-and-burlapped. Never buy bareroot magnolias. Pick a site in full sun that is 12' or more from other trees or buildings. Dig a hole at least 18" deep and twice as wide as the root ball. Set the plant so it's a little higher than it was at the nursery. Refill the hole with a mixture of equal parts soil and peat moss, rotted manure, or compost. Firm the soil around the rootball, then scrape excess soil away from the plant to form a shallow basin for holding water. Thoroughly soak the soil with water.

After planting, spread a 3" layer of organic mulch over top. Add new material as the mulch decomposes. Rainfall usually provides enough water for magnolias. In very dry areas, however, you should soak the soil once a week. If your magnolia shows signs of malnutrition—small, pale, sparse leaves or short twig growth—you can apply lawn fertilizer in late fall or early spring. Use 2 pounds per inch of trunk diameter. Spread the fertilizer around the tree in a 2' to 3' wide band beneath the branches. Water it into the soil.

Late spring is the best time to prune magnolias. Coat all wounds with a good-quality paint or a commercial tree-wound dressing.

S hrubs are inexpensive, almost care-free, and come in a wide variety to choose from. They produce flowers from early spring until the snow flies, and cover a large area with the least number of plants than any other group in Mother Nature's kingdom. There are shrubs for damp spots, wet spots, shaded areas, full sun, clay soil, sand and, yes, even gravel. There are shrubs for privacy screens, hedges, group plantings or ones that look beautiful just standing alone. There are shrubs that provide flowers, foliage, fruit and willowy beauty when they are bare of leaves in the winter snows. In short, there's a shrub for everyone and every one occasion.

To get the most out of your shrubs, you must take a few precautions. First, ask yourself what do you expect your shrub to do? For instance, if you want to direct traffic, you would not ask a flowering almond to withstand the rush of homeward bound school children.

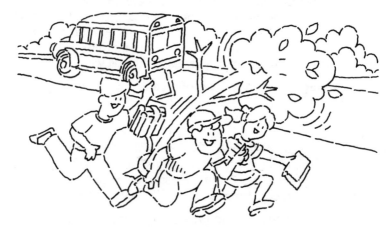

That's a job designed for Mr. Barberry (he is qualified and more to the point; ouch!) You wouldn't ask my fragrant friend, Miss Lilac, to absorb a damp situation you had in a low spot. After all, she prefers high ground. That "damp job" is best handled by the Red Twig Dogwood.

FLOWERING SHRUBS

Flowering shrubs are the best friends a gardener ever had. They are, by far and away, the most beautiful, fragrant and economical garden plants. They need the least amount of care, adapt to almost any location, provide a wide assortment of colors, sizes, and shapes, and offer the most value for the money. They are often overlooked and dug out by some green thumbers who want a no-maintenance garden.

Planting shrubs requires a minimum of preparation; just plant them the day of purchase, make the hole twice as large as necessary, and only as deep as in the nursery; mix the removed soil with gypsum; and lastly, mulch them with a good 2" of wood chips.

HINTS FOR SELECTION

You must use a little discretion in your selection. Remember this: plan before you plant. Take the layout you made of your yard and design the areas you want to plant in. Review the mail order catalogs and check nursery plant tags for important information—your nursery person is also a prime reference source. You can learn about the amount of sun, soil and drainage required, how tall and wide certain shrubs grow, when they bloom and flower and in what color, whether they foliate after blooming, and blossom with or without fragrance, and whether they produce edible or ornamental berries or fruit.

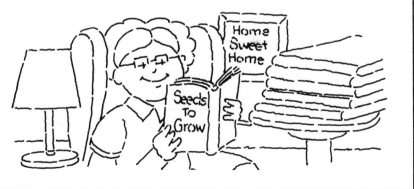

America's / Master Gardener®

⚘ SHRUBS

This knowledge will help you to grow a healthy yarden alive with radiant color; you'll also be aware of the pitfalls of over-planting (like root crowding) and misplanting (as bedding acid-loving shrubs with those requiring neutral soil).

PLANTING

In the colder climates, early spring is the best time to plant shrubs. In the mild climate zones, plant in either spring or fall. In the southern regions, planting can be done whenever plants are available. (You lucky dogs, you!)

Follow these simple steps (which should be almost second nature by now) for planting:

1. Dig the planting hole twice as large, and 1" deeper than the one the plant was growing in at the nursery.
2. Add 1 handful of bonemeal and 2 handsful of gypsum to the soil when planting.
3. Cover the soil with 2 or 3 layers of newspaper and cover the newspaper with mulch.
4. Spray all newly-planted shrubs with a mild fruit tree solution to discourage insects from visiting.

WATERING

Water shrubs daily for 3 to 4 days immediately after planting. As soon as a plant is established, a weekly soaking will do. It is best to use a soaker hose rather than a sprinkler or nozzle.

PRUNING

Shrubs that bloom in spring should only be pruned right after they bloom. Summer blooming shrubs should be pruned in early spring. When pruning, always cut just above a bud or branch that is growing to the outside, or in the direction you want the new growth to follow. Always use sharp, clean tools and seal any cut larger than your little finger with a mixture of antiseptic mouthwash and latex paint.

WEED CONTROL

It is a good idea to avoid excessive cultivation underneath shrubs. Any one of the many attractive groundcovers can be used. Weeds that appear can be destroyed with any of the available weed controls.

FEEDING

Do not feed shrubs immediately after planting; wait at least 4 weeks. Since most shrubs are not meant to grow more than 10' to 12' high, a well-balanced garden food (5-10-10) can be applied in early spring in most parts of the county, and in both fall and spring in the southern regions. Do not let dry fertilizers come in contact with roots. Shrubs can be fed also with tree spikes or a root feeder.

MAINTENANCE

Begin with an early spring shower of liquid dish soap and water (1 cup to 20 gallons), then dormant spray as soon as the weather permits. Mulch the soil beneath the shrubs with 2" of shredded bark or wood chips, apply paradichlorobenzene on the soil, and mulch to destroy borers and other ground insects. Pour 5 pounds of gypsum per plant onto the soil to loosen and condition it for more effective fertilizer action. A low-nitrogen type nutrient can be applied once in early March (before bloom) and again in June (after bloom).

Liquid dish soap, chewing tobacco juice and antiseptic mouthwash should be the only preventative spray that you use on your yarden. Insecticides should be used only when a problem arises; then isolate the cause and apply the appropriate chemical at the recommended rate and for the specified period. I have found that a liquid combination spray containing Malathion, Sevin or Captan is about the safest for me and my plants.

INSECT AND DISEASE CONTROL

I have found that applying Dursban to the soil and an all-purpose fruit & garden spray to the foliage in both spring and fall will just about insure complete control.

America's / Master Gardener*

MAKING YOUR OWN CUTTINGS

Softwood cuttings are slips of plants that are taken from the adult plant's soft growth. Most of your perennials and flowering shrubs will yield these cuttings. Take your cuttings in May and early June from new growth. Make the cutting 3" to 6" long, and remove the bottom 3 layers of leaves. Dip them first into water, then about 1/2" into a product called Rootone. Shake off the excess and place in a pre-poked, pencil sized hole in your rooting material (sharp sand), covering at least 1 or 2 of the nodes (leaf breaks). The best temperature for rooting is 60° to 70°F, while the soil should be 5° warmer. Keep the soil shaded and always damp, but not soaked for the first few days. Sprinkle the foliage often to control humidity.

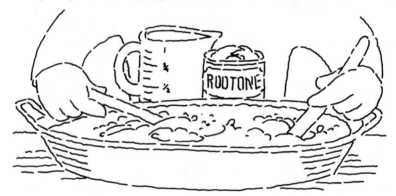

Move the cuttings into the light as they start rooting. When roots are well established, pot them up and move them into the garden. Plant the cuttings, pots and all, into the soil to protect them.

Hardwood cuttings are collected in late fall or winter. Cut them 6" to 8" long, tie in bundles, and store in a box of peat moss in the basement until spring. After the threat of frost is past, remove them, dip in Rootone, and then place the slips into the soil in your garden, leaving about half of the stem above the ground. That's all there is to it!

GROUNDCOVERS

The variety of climbing vines and creeping groundcovers is virtually unlimited as far as color, texture and fragrance is concerned. Both vines and groundcovers are nearly maintenance-free, with a few exceptions. And both tend to produce new plants without much effort.

THE UPS AND DOWNS

Whenever anyone thinks of a climbing vine, they naturally think of a flowering vine. But since we're all concerned about space in this day and age, we should first consider a plant that will return both food and flowers. When it is necessary to disguise an object or location, I always look at my fruit and vegetable list first. There are many vinelike crops such as pole beans, peas, grape vines, etc. that can do the job and pay their way at the same time. If it is a groundcover that I need, I always check to see if strawberries, cucumbers, or squash will fill the bill. Don't waste space if you can fill your table and eye at the same time.

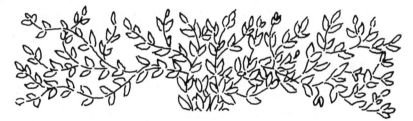

When you select a vine for flowers and/or foliage, it should serve some purpose. The plant can be used to detract from an objectionable surface, perhaps a crumbling or stained wall. In that case, the plant should be trained to grow on wires to form a design.

To make an arbor, you should use a dense foliage vine with delicate flowers. If you want to divide your yard into recreational areas, you can use medium foliage vines with large flowers, etc. Entryways can be enhanced by using cascading vines like the wisteria, to give the effect of elegance and size. Before you select a vine, however, decide what its purpose in life is going to be.

Jerry Baker
America's Master Gardener®

🐌 GROUNDCOVERS

NO MAN'S LAND

Anyone who has attempted to grow grass under trees, or in heavily shaded areas, is fighting a losing battle for both himself and the grass. Groundcovers are the answer to your grass' prayers and your problems. These hardy boys can manage almost any situation: shade, partial shade, damp, wet or soggy soil. The groundcover crowd lives by the popular old saying, "When the going gets tough, the tough get going!"

Vines and groundcovers are tough customers, but only after they've established themselves in their new homes. Spade leaf mulch, peat moss, and garden food into the soil where you are going to plant your climbers or crawlers. Make sure the soil is the same as for the vegetable garden—level and fine. I plant them rather close together, in staggered rows. Top-dress the soil with a regular garden food at least twice a year.

Most groundcovers are virtually indestructible. Since they grow like weeds, I plant my groundcovers in May when weeds are growing best. This is a good time anyplace in the country.

KEEPING BUGS OUT

You will find that you are not the only one that appreciates a thick cover of green foliage. Almost every bug in your yarden will, at one time or another, stop by to rest in it. Mice and moles will occasionally take a breather or build a winter nest there. To discourage insects, bathe your groundcovers at least once a month with this tonic in your 20 gal. hose-end sprayer:

1 cup liquid dish soap

1 cup chewing tobacco juice

1 cup antiseptic mouthwash

fill the balance of the sprayer jar with warm water

To control soil bugs, use dry Dursban at the recommended rate.

WEEDS

Weeds shouldn't be a problem if you use one of the "kneeless weeder controls" in early spring. I do not cultivate groundcovers, but I do mulch after I have applied the kneeless weeder. Otherwise, the thick foliage should keep just about all but the most stubborn uninvited guests out.

SUPPORT YOUR LOYAL VINES

Vines are much heavier than you can imagine. Make sure that the supporting pole or post is well anchored, and the wires are thick and tough. Vines can usually hold on tight to whatever you supply: some have fine roots like fingers (especially the ivies), while grapes wrap their fingers around anything in sight. Some twist their whole body around a wire or pole (like bittersweet), while still others have sticky fingers to help them hold on.

WHO'S WHO

The following is a brief list of who's who in the climber and creeper crowd. For more information, check out the mail order catalogues you collected to help you with your landscaping.

Climbers
- Wisteria • Clematis (princess of the garden) • Star Jasmine
- Trumpet Vine • Boston Ivy • Winter Creeper (Scale's Delight)
- Passion Flower • Fatshedera • Morning Glory • English Ivy
- Flame Honeysuckle • Common Honeysuckle • Bougainvillea
- Vine Lilac • Madeiravine • Pyracantha (living barbed wire)
- Silver Lace Vine • Climbing Hydrangea • Waxy Bittersweet
(looks great in a vase)

Creepers
- Bishop's Weed • Carpet Bugle • Chamomile (makes a nice tea as well) • Crownvetch • Sedum • Winter Creeper (Colorata)
- Hardy Baltic Ivy • Myrtle

America's / Master Gardener®

CONVERSION
Table

MULTIPLY	TO OBTAIN
Feet by 30.48	Centimeters
Feet by .3048	Meter
Gallons by 3.785	Liter
Gallons Water by 8.3453	Lbs. of Water
Inches by 2.540	Centimeter
Meters by 3.281	Feet
Meters by 39.37	Inches
Miles by 1.609	Kilometer
Miles Per Hr. by 1.609	Kilometers Per Hr.
Millimeters by 0.03937	Inches
Ounces by 2	Tablespoons (Liq.)
Ounces by 6	Teaspoons (Liq.)
Ounces by 3	Tablespoons (Dry)
Ounces by 9	Teaspoons (Dry)
Tablespoons (Liq.) by 0.5	Ounce
Tablespoons (Dry) by 0.3333	Ounce
Temp (C) +17.78 by 1.8	Temp (F)
Temp (F) -32 by 5/9	Temp (C)

LIQUID VOLUME EQUIVALENTS

Gal.	Qt.	Pt.	Fl. Oz.	Cups	Tbsp.	Tsp.
1	4	8	128	16		
	1	2	32	4		
		1	16	2	32	
			1	1/8	2	6
				1	16	48
					1	3
						1

TURF MEASUREMENT

1 acre ....43,560 sq. ft.